Cancer Cookbook for Beginners

The Complete Cancer Diet Guide with Essential Nutritious Whole Food Anti-Cancer Recipes for Treatment & Recovery

copyrighted@2023

John Elena

Table of Contents

Chapter One

Introduction to Cancer Diet
Understanding the Role of Nutrition in Cancer

In the complex tapestry of cancer treatment, the importance of nutrition cannot be overstated. The journey through cancer is not only a battle of medical interventions, but also a daily commitment to nourish the body with the right nutrients. It serves as a compass to guide the reader through the basic principles underlying the relationship between nutrition and cancer.

The Power of Nutrient-Dense Foods:

The foundation of an effective anti-cancer diet is a commitment to include nutrient-dense foods. We explore the key role that vitamins, minerals and other essential nutrients play in supporting the body's natural defenses. From immune system function to cellular repair, every bite consumed has the potential to be a building block for recovery.

Antioxidants: Nature's Defense Mechanism:

We'll delve into the science behind antioxidants and uncover their essential role in neutralizing free radicals that can damage cells and DNA. By understanding the sources of these powerful compounds, readers will gain insight into how to use the abundance of antioxidant-rich fruits, vegetables, and other plant foods to promote healing and resilience.

Essential Vitamins and Minerals:

This section serves as a practical guide to the vitamins and minerals that are particularly important in cancer treatment. From the immune-boosting properties of vitamin C to the bone-strengthening benefits of vitamin D, we demystify the alphabet soup of essential nutrients and empower readers to make informed, targeted dietary decisions.

Balancing Act: Proteins, Carbohydrates and Fats:

Cancer treatment can place unique demands on the body's energy and nutritional requirements. In this segment, we explore the delicate balance between protein, carbohydrates and fat and offer insight into how this balance can be tailored to individual needs. Achieving the right balance is key, whether it's building muscle, maintaining energy levels or promoting overall well-being.

Hydration: Fuel for regeneration:

Often overlooked, hydration is the cornerstone of a healthy cancer diet. We shed light on the importance of adequate water intake and explored how staying hydrated can reduce common treatment side effects, aid digestion and contribute to an overall sense of vitality.

The Importance of a Well-Balanced Diet during Cancer Treatment

Embarking on the journey of cancer treatment comes with countless challenges, and one of the most impressive ways to navigate this journey is by adopting a well-balanced and nutritious diet. In this section, we will highlight the critical role that a thoughtfully designed diet plays in supporting the body and mind during cancer treatment trials.

Nutrition for Resilience:

A properly balanced diet serves as a cornerstone of resilience during cancer treatment. The body goes through a series of physical and emotional stressors, and proper nutrition becomes a powerful tool for strengthening. By providing the necessary nutrients, a balanced diet supports the body's ability to cope with the demands of treatment, promoting a sense of strength and endurance.

Sustainable Energy Level:

Cancer treatments such as chemotherapy and radiation can often lead to fatigue and decreased energy levels. A well-balanced diet provides a steady supply of energy helps individuals maintain their daily activities and, just as importantly, supports the body's natural healing processes. A strategic combination of carbohydrates, proteins and healthy fats becomes a source of lasting vitality.

Construction and Repair Fabrics:

Cancer treatment can affect the body at the cellular level, requiring tissue repair and remodeling. Adequate protein intake becomes instrumental in this process, as proteins are the building blocks of cells and tissues. We explore how a well-balanced diet rich in lean protein contributes to cell repair and helps on the road to recovery.

Strengthening Immunity:

Maintaining a strong immune system is paramount in cancer treatment. The interplay of vitamins, minerals and antioxidants in a balanced diet plays a key role in strengthening the body's natural defense mechanisms. By understanding the immune-boosting properties of various foods, individuals can take an active role in strengthening their resistance to infection and promoting overall health.

Management of Side Effects:

Side effects of cancer treatment, such as nausea, changes in taste, and fluctuations in appetite, can significantly affect nutrient intake. A well-balanced diet takes these challenges into account and offers strategies and recipes that are not only nutritionally dense, but also tailored to address specific side effects and ensure that individuals get the nutrition they need, even when they face obstacles.

Improving the Quality of Life:

In addition to the physiological benefits, a well-balanced diet contributes to improving the quality of life. The enjoyment of eating tasty and satisfying foods can positively impact emotional well-being and provide comfort and joy during a challenging time. We explore the psychological dimensions of food and emphasize the importance of culinary enjoyment in promoting positive thinking.

Chapter Two

Nourishing Your Body
Nutrient-Rich Foods for Cancer Patients

In the complex tapestry of cancer treatment, the role of nutrient-dense foods is becoming paramount. These foods serve as the foundation for a resilient, well-nourished body and provide the essential building blocks needed to combat the challenges of cancer. This section explores a spectrum of nutrient-dense options, each selected for their unique contribution to overall well-being.

1. Colorful vegetables and fruits:

   - Vibrant, colorful vegetables and fruits are a treasure trove of vitamins, minerals and antioxidants. From beta-carotene in carrots to vitamin C in berries, each shade means a different set of health benefits. We dive into the rainbow of possibilities and offer creative ways to incorporate these cancer-fighting foods into everyday meals.

2. Leafy greens:

   - Swiss chard, kale, and other dark, leafy greens are nutrient-dense powerhouses. Full of vitamins A, C and K, as well as minerals such as iron and calcium, this vegetable helps support immunity, bone health and overall vitality. Recipes and ideas for incorporating these leafy wonders into everyday meals take center stage.

3. Whole Grains:

   - Whole grains are a rich source of fiber, antioxidants and essential nutrients. Quinoa, brown rice, and oats feature prominently in this section, offering not only sustained energy, but also contributing to digestive health. Easy-to-follow recipes show the versatility of whole grains in creating healthy and satisfying meals.

4. Lean proteins:

   - Protein is the cornerstone for cell repair and regeneration. The focus is on lean sources such as poultry, fish, tofu and legumes, which provide essential amino acids without unnecessary saturated fat. The recipes focus on creating protein-rich dishes that are nutritious and delicious.

5. Healthy Fats:

   - Omega-3 fatty acids found in fatty fish, flaxseeds and walnuts play a vital role in reducing inflammation and heart health.

We explore the world of healthy fats, dispel myths and provide practical suggestions on how to incorporate them into your diet. The recipes showcase the wonderful combination of taste and health in dishes rich in these essential fats.

6. Dairy products or dairy alternatives:

   - Dairy products and fortified milk alternatives contribute to the intake of calcium and vitamin D, which are vital for bone health. This outlines options for those who may be lactose intolerant or prefer non-dairy alternatives. From smoothies to savory dishes, the focus is on maintaining a calcium-rich diet without compromising on taste.

7. Hydrating foods:

   - In addition to drinks, certain foods contribute significantly to hydration. Water-rich fruits and vegetables like cucumbers, watermelon, and oranges are being researched for their dual benefits of hydration and nutrient content. We share practical tips for incorporating these foods into your daily meals.

Navigating the vast array of nutrient-dense foods isn't just about nutrition; it's about making a deliberate choice to strengthen the body's fight against cancer. By understanding and embracing the diversity of these foods, individuals can develop a taste for healing and resilience, one delicious and nutritious bite at a time.

The Power of Antioxidants in the Fight against Cancer

Cancer, a complex and often formidable adversary, prompts the search for different strategies to support the body's defenses. Among these strategies, the power of antioxidants is emerging as a key player in the fight against cancer. Antioxidants are compounds that neutralize free radicals—unstable molecules that, if left unchecked, can damage cells and contribute to the development and progression of cancer. Here's a closer look at the profound effects of antioxidants in cancer:

1. Neutralization of free radicals:

   - Free radicals are produced naturally in the body during various metabolic processes. Additionally, exposure to environmental factors such as pollution, radiation, and tobacco smoke can increase the production of free radicals. These molecules with unpaired electrons seek stability by stealing electrons from other molecules, causing a chain reaction that can lead to cell damage. Antioxidants intervene by donating electrons to neutralize free radicals and stop this potentially harmful cascade.

2. Protection of cellular DNA:

   - The DNA in our cells is a critical target for free radical damage. When free radicals interact with DNA, mutations can occur that potentially trigger the initiation and progression of cancer. Antioxidants help protect the integrity of DNA by preventing these harmful interactions and contributing to the maintenance of healthy cells.

3. Anti-inflammatory effects:

- One known factor in the development of cancer is chronic inflammation. Antioxidants, especially those found in fruits, vegetables and spices, have anti-inflammatory properties. By reducing inflammation, antioxidants create an environment less favorable for cancer cells to grow and spread.

4. Strengthening immune function:

- A robust immune system is crucial in identifying and killing cancer cells. Antioxidants support immune function by reducing oxidative stress, which can compromise the effectiveness of immune responses. By supporting a balanced immune environment, antioxidants contribute to the body's ability to recognize and fight abnormal cell growth.

5. Apoptosis and death of cancer cells:

   - Apoptosis, programmed cell death, is a natural process that eliminates damaged or abnormal cells. Cancer cells often evade apoptosis, which allows them to proliferate. Some antioxidants have been found to induce apoptosis in cancer cells, promoting their elimination and preventing further growth.

6. DNA Repair and Maintenance:

   - Antioxidants play a role in DNA repair mechanisms. When cells are exposed to oxidative stress, antioxidants help repair DNA damage and prevent the accumulation of mutations that could contribute to the development of cancer. This proactive maintenance supports the overall health of the cellular environment.

7. Complementary treatment support:

- Although not a stand-alone cancer treatment, antioxidants can complement traditional cancer treatments. Some studies suggest that antioxidants may increase the effectiveness of some cancer treatments, reduce side effects, and contribute to overall well-being during treatment.

It is important to note that the relationship between antioxidants and cancer is complex and not all studies provide conclusive evidence. The effectiveness of antioxidants can depend on factors such as the type of cancer, the specific antioxidants involved, and the individual's health status.

Essential Vitamins and Minerals

In the complex tapestry of cancer treatment, the role of vitamins and minerals is similar to the warp and weft that form the basis for the body's resilience and recovery. This section examines the essential vitamins and minerals that are crucial for individuals undergoing cancer treatment and highlights their specific contribution to overall well-being.

1. Vitamin C:

- Functions: Vitamin C, known for its immune properties, plays a vital role in collagen synthesis, wound healing and antioxidant defense. Increases the absorption of non-heme iron, crucial for individuals with anemia.

- Sources: Citrus fruits, strawberries, peppers, broccoli, kiwi.

2. Vitamin D:

- Function: Essential for bone health, vitamin D aids in the absorption of calcium and phosphorus. In addition, it contributes to immune function and can have anti-inflammatory effects.

   - Sources: Sunlight, fatty fish (e.g. salmon, mackerel), fortified dairy products, eggs.

3. Vitamin E:

   - Functions: A powerful antioxidant, vitamin E protects cells from oxidative damage. It supports immune function and may have anti-inflammatory effects.

   - Sources: Nuts (especially almonds), seeds (sunflower seeds), spinach, broccoli, vegetable oils.

4. Vitamin A:

- Functions: Important for vision, immune function and skin health, vitamin A is also an antioxidant. Its precursor, beta-carotene, is converted into vitamin A in the body.

- Sources: Sweet potatoes, carrots, cabbage, spinach, liver, eggs.

5. Vitamin K:

- Functions: Vitamin K is essential for blood clotting and bone metabolism, it also plays a role in regulating blood calcium levels.

- Sources: Leafy vegetables (cabbage, spinach, collards),

broccoli, Brussels sprouts, fish, meat.

6. B vitamins (B6, B12, folic acid):

   - Functions: These vitamins play a key role in energy metabolism, DNA synthesis and red blood cell formation. Folate is especially important for preventing neural tube defects during pregnancy.

   - Sources: B6 - bananas, poultry, fish; B12 - meat, dairy products, eggs; Folate - leafy greens, legumes, fortified cereals.

7. Calcium:

- Functions: Calcium is vital for bone health and nerve function, it also plays a role in muscle contraction and blood clotting.

- Sources: Dairy products, fortified vegetable milk, leafy greens, almonds, tofu.

8. Iron:

- Function: Iron is necessary for the transport of oxygen in the blood, it is part of hemoglobin. Adequate iron intake is essential to prevent anemia.

- Sources: Red meat, poultry, fish, beans, lentils, fortified cereals.

9. Zinc:

- Functions: Zinc, a component of enzymes involved in immune function and wound healing, also supports DNA synthesis.

- Sources: Meat, dairy products, nuts, seeds, legumes.

10. Magnesium:

- Functions: Involved in muscle and nerve function, blood glucose control and bone health, magnesium also plays a role in energy metabolism.

- Sources: Leafy greens, nuts, seeds, whole grains, legumes.

Understanding the importance of these vitamins and minerals provides a blueprint for creating a diet that supports overall health during cancer treatment. However, individual nutritional needs may vary and consultation with healthcare professionals is recommended to tailor dietary choices to specific medical conditions and treatment plans. A symphony of vitamins and minerals, when harmoniously incorporated into a well-balanced diet, becomes a powerful ally on the road to resilience and recovery.

Chapter Three

Building a Foundation
Creating a Plaque to Fight Cancer

Making a cancer board is an art that involves harmonizing different nutrients to help the body fight cancer. This explores the principles and practical steps for putting together meals that not only provide nutrition but also contribute to overall well-being.

1. Colorful vegetables as a base:

   - Start by filling at least half of your plate with a varied palette of colorful vegetables. Different colors mean different nutrients and antioxidants. Dark leafy greens, cruciferous vegetables and a spectrum of hues provide a variety of vitamins and minerals essential to support immunity and overall health.

2. Lean Proteins for Cell Repair:

   - Allocate a quarter of your plate to lean protein. Whether from poultry, fish, tofu, legumes or plant sources, protein is the building block for cellular repair and regeneration. Choose grilled, baked or sautéed to maintain nutritional integrity.

3. Whole grains for sustained energy:

- Devote another quarter of your plate to whole grain products. Options like quinoa, brown rice, or whole wheat provide complex carbohydrates that slowly release energy and promote sustained vitality. These grains also offer fiber, which supports digestion and contributes to a feeling of fullness.

4. Healthy Fats for Nutrient Absorption:

- Integrate healthy fats into your plate to improve the absorption of fat-soluble vitamins. Avocado slices, nuts, seeds or a drop of olive oil not only add flavor, but also bring essential fatty acids to the table. Pay attention to portions, focus on quality fat sources.

5. Hydrating foods for balance:

- Fill your plate with hydrating foods like cucumber, watermelon or celery. These not only contribute to overall hydration, but also supply additional vitamins and minerals. Consider incorporating hydrating foods into salads, snacks, or as a side dish.

6. Mindful Portion Control:

- Take care when determining how much food to eat. Be attuned to your hunger and fullness signals and allow your body to guide your eating habits. Consider using smaller plates to create a visually satisfying meal while naturally moderating portion sizes.

7. Culinary herbs and spices for taste and health:

   - Boost the nutritional profile and flavor of your plate with culinary herbs and spices. In addition to adding zest, many herbs and spices have anti-inflammatory and antioxidant properties. Experiment with fresh herbs like basil, cilantro or mint and spices like turmeric, ginger and garlic.

8. Whole, unprocessed foods:

- Favor whole, unprocessed foods over their refined counterparts. Fresh, minimally processed ingredients retain their nutritional value and provide a spectrum of vitamins, minerals and phytonutrients essential for immune function and overall health.

9. Balanced combinations for variety:

   - Create balanced and varied combinations to provide a wide range of nutrients. Rotate your choices regularly to introduce variety, both in terms of taste and nutrition. This not only promotes overall health, but also keeps meals interesting and enjoyable.

Remember that this is a guideline rather than a strict prescription. Modifications can be made based on individual preferences, dietary restrictions and nutritional needs. The goal is to build a plate that is not only visually appealing, but also a source of nutrients, supports the body's resistance and strengthens its defenses in the face of cancer.

Balance of Proteins, Carbohydrates and Fats

Achieving a harmonious balance between proteins, carbohydrates and fats is a key element in creating a complete and nutritious diet, especially during cancer treatment. This explores the different roles of each macronutrient and provides practical insights into achieving the right balance tailored to individual needs.

1. The role of proteins:

   - Function: The building blocks of all cells, tissues, and organs are proteins. During cancer treatment, they play a vital role in cell repair, immune function and overall resistance.

   - Sources: Lean meat, poultry, fish, eggs, dairy products, legumes, tofu and plant-based protein sources such as quinoa and lentils.

2. Importance of Carbohydrates:

   - Function: The body uses carbs as its main energy source. Optimum intake of carbohydrates ensures constant and permanent release of energy supports daily activities and overall vitality.

- Sources: Whole grains (brown rice, quinoa, whole wheat), fruits, vegetables and legumes.

3. Healthy Fats for Nutrient Absorption:

- Function: Fats are essential for the absorption of nutrients, especially fat-soluble vitamins A, D, E and K. They also provide a concentrated source of energy and play a role in the structure of the cell membrane.

- Sources: Avocado, nuts, seeds, olive oil, fatty fish (salmon, mackerel) and flax seeds.

4. Finding the right balance of proteins, carbohydrates and fats:

   - The ideal balance of macronutrients may vary depending on individual health conditions, treatment regimens and personal preferences. While there is no one-size-fits-all ratio, a balanced plate typically includes:

   - Protein: 25-30% of total calories.

   - Carbohydrates: 45-60% of total calories, with an emphasis on complex carbohydrates.

- Fats: 20-35% of total calories, with a focus on healthy fats.

5. Sewing for individual needs:

- Individual nutritional needs may vary and adjustments should be made based on factors such as weight, activity level and treatment side effects. Some individuals may benefit from a higher protein intake, while others may require adjustment of carbohydrate sources based on digestive sensitivity.

6. Protein Packed Options for Cancer Patients:

- For those undergoing cancer treatment, it is essential to incorporate easily digestible sources of protein. Options like yogurt, eggs, smoothies with protein powder, and small, frequent meals can help meet protein needs without taxing the digestive system.

7. Complex Carbohydrates for Sustained Energy:

- Favor complex carbohydrates such as whole grains and legumes to ensure a sustained release of energy. These sources also offer fiber, which supports digestive health and prevents energy spikes and crashes.

8. Healthy fats for overall well-being:

   - Include sources of healthy fats in your diet to promote overall well-being. Avocado, nuts and olive oil not only contribute to the absorption of nutrients, but also add flavor and satiety to meals.

9. Practical tips for balancing:

   - Experiment with portion sizes and ratios to see what works best for you.

   - Include a variety of foods to ensure a varied intake of nutrients.

- Pay attention to your body's cues of hunger and fullness.

10. Consultation with healthcare professionals:

- For individuals with specific dietary or health concerns, consultation with health professionals, including registered dietitians, is essential. They can provide personalized counseling and ensure nutritional needs are met during the challenges of cancer treatment.

Hydration and its Effect on Healing

In the complex dance of healing, hydration is emerging as a

cornerstone for overall well-being, especially in the challenging environment of cancer treatment. This explores the essential role of hydration, its impact on the healing process, and practical strategies for maintaining optimal fluid balance.

1. The importance of adequate hydration:

   - Proper hydration is the basis for supporting the body's physiological functions. During cancer treatment, maintaining adequate fluid balance is even more important, as hydration plays a role in mitigating side effects, supporting immune function, and contributing to overall vitality.

2. Mitigation of treatment side effects:

   - Many cancer treatments, such as chemotherapy and radiation, can cause side effects such as nausea, vomiting, and diarrhea. Adequate hydration helps alleviate these symptoms by ensuring the body stays hydrated, reducing the severity of side effects and promoting a more comfortable treatment experience.

3. Support of immune function:

- Hydration is closely linked to immune function. Proper fluid balance ensures that immune cells can move freely throughout the body and effectively watch for and respond to abnormal cells. Staying hydrated is a proactive way to strengthen the body's natural defenses during the healing process.

4. Facilitation of nutrient transport:

   - Nutrients important for healing, such as vitamins and minerals, are transported through the bloodstream. Optimal hydration ensures efficient transport of nutrients into cells, supports cell repair, regeneration and the overall recovery process.

5. Improving digestive function:

   - Hydration plays a key role in maintaining the health of the digestive tract. It helps with digestion and absorption of nutrients, prevents constipation and promotes overall gastrointestinal well-being. This is especially important in cancer treatment, as digestive problems are a common side effect.

6. Strategies for Staying Hydrated:

   - Regular water intake: Aim for at least 8 cups (64 ounces) of water per day, adjusted according to individual needs and treatment side effects.

- Infused Water: Add natural flavors to your water with slices of citrus fruits, berries or herbs to make hydration more attractive.

- Herbal teas: Decaffeinated herbal teas promote fluid intake and provide additional benefits such as soothing properties or antioxidant content.

- Hydrating foods: Include water-rich foods like watermelon, cucumber, and oranges in your meals and snacks.

- Small, frequent sips: Rather than large amounts at once, encourage small, frequent sips throughout the day to improve fluid absorption.

7. Monitoring the state of hydration:

- Watch for signs of dehydration such as dark urine, dizziness or dry mouth. If fluid intake is difficult due to side effects of treatment, consult with your health care professional for guidance on maintaining optimal hydration levels.

8. Individual Hydration Plans:

- Hydration needs may vary depending on factors such as age, weight, climate and type of treatment. Individual hydration plans, developed in consultation with healthcare professionals, ensure that specific needs are met to support the healing journey.

9. Hydration as a self-care ritual:

- Viewing hydration as a conscious and intentional act of self-care can shift the perspective from a mere task to a caring practice. Taking a moment to enjoy a refreshing glass of water or herbal tea can become a ritual that contributes not only to physical well-being, but also to mental and emotional resilience.

As a cornerstone of health and healing, hydration becomes a proactive and empowering tool during cancer treatment. By prioritizing fluid balance, individuals embark on a journey that not only supports the body's complex healing processes, but also promotes a sense of vitality and well-being in the face of adversity.

Chapter Four

Medicinal Cuisine

Midway through the cancer journey, the kitchen turns into a sanctuary of healing. This section delves into the therapeutic properties of culinary herbs, spices, and nutrient-dense foods and guides readers through the art of creating foods that not only nourish the body, but also contribute to the overall healing process. From the anti-inflammatory magic of turmeric to the digestive support of ginger, this section explores the healing properties of ingredients that elevate the kitchen to a space of resilience and well-being.

1. Turmeric: The Golden Anti-Inflammatory Powerhouse

   - Properties: Known for its active compound, curcumin, turmeric has powerful anti-inflammatory and antioxidant properties.

   - In the kitchen: Explore recipes for golden turmeric lattes, curries, and soups that showcase the versatility of this healing spice.

2. Ginger: A soothing digestive symphony

- Properties: Ginger offers anti-nausea and anti-inflammatory effects, making it a soothing companion for digestive health.

- In the kitchen: Discover the warmth of ginger in teas, stir-fries and ginger broths designed to aid digestion.

3. Garlic: Immunity-boosting elixir

- Properties: In addition to its culinary charm, garlic is celebrated for its immune and antibacterial properties.

- In the kitchen: From roasted garlic spreads to garlic-infused olive oils, explore ways to incorporate this aromatic bulb into everyday meals.

4. Cinnamon: Balancing Blood Sugar and more

   - Properties: Not only does cinnamon add sweetness without sugar, but it also helps balance blood sugar levels and offers antioxidant benefits.

   - In the kitchen: Indulge in the soothing aroma of cinnamon in oatmeal, smoothies and baked goods for a delicious and healthy twist.

5. Mint: Cooling and refreshing digestion

- Features: The cooling properties of mint make it a refreshing choice for digestive support and a pleasant addition to drinks.

- In the kitchen: From mint water to salads and desserts, explore the invigorating essence of this herb.

6. Rosemary: Supports memory and circulation

- Properties: Rosemary not only enhances culinary creations, but also offers potential cognitive and circulatory benefits.

- In the kitchen: Elevate dishes with rosemary oils, roasted vegetables and hearty stews that showcase their aromatic richness.

7. Berries: Antioxidant-packed delight

   - Properties: Berries with their vibrant colors are rich in antioxidants, promote overall health and potentially help prevent cancer.

- In the kitchen: Explore the sweetness of berries in smoothies, salads and desserts that deliver an explosion of flavor and nutrition.

8. Salmon: A culinary elixir rich in Omega-3

   - Properties: Fatty fish such as salmon, rich in omega-3 fatty acids, contribute to reduced inflammation and heart health.

   - In the kitchen: Enjoy the flavors of grilled or baked salmon, discover marinades and side dishes that showcase its nutritional capabilities.

9. Dark leafy greens: Increase in nutrient content

   - Properties: Cabbage, spinach and other dark leafy vegetables are nutritional sources that offer a spectrum of vitamins and minerals.

- In the kitchen: Incorporate this vegetable into salads, smoothies and sautés for a nutrient boost.

10. Medicinal elixirs: Teas, broths and infusions

- Properties: In addition to individual ingredients, the chapter explores the creation of healing elixirs, including herbal teas, nourishing broths, and infused waters.

- In the kitchen: Immerse yourself in recipes that combine various healing elements to create drinks that soothe, rejuvenate and contribute to overall well-being.

Recipes for Strength and Regeneration

Breakfast Boosters: Energizing Appetizers

Starting the day with a nutritious and energizing breakfast is a cornerstone for individuals undergoing cancer treatment. It focuses on breakfast recipes that not only provide essential nutrients, but also offer a pleasant and uplifting start to the day. From hearty oatmeal bowls to energizing smoothie bowls, these recipes are created to nourish the body, promote sustained energy, and set a positive tone for the day ahead.

1. Nut Banana Oatmeal:

   - Ingredients: Oatmeal, almond milk, bananas, nut butter, chia seeds.

   - Benefits: A convenient and nutrient-packed breakfast rich in fiber, healthy fats and energy-sustaining carbohydrates.

2. Energizing Green Smoothie Bowl:

   - Ingredients: spinach, pineapple, banana, Greek yogurt, almond milk, toppings (granola, chia seeds, forest fruits).

   - Benefits: A vibrant and antioxidant-rich smoothie bowl to start the day with a burst of energy and essential nutrients.

3. Apple Cinnamon Quinoa Porridge:

   - Ingredients: Quinoa, apples, cinnamon, almond milk, honey.

   - Benefits: Warm and comforting porridge containing quinoa for protein, apples for fiber and cinnamon for added flavor and potential blood sugar balance.

4. Breakfast toast with avocado and tomatoes:

  - Ingredients: Whole grain bread, avocado, cherry tomatoes, feta cheese, olive oil.

  - Benefits: A salty and nutrient-rich breakfast with beneficial fats from avocado and the freshness of tomatoes.

5. Smoothie with strawberry and almond butter:

  - Ingredients: Mixed berries, almond butter, Greek yogurt, almond milk, honey.

  - Benefits: A delicious protein-rich smoothie that supports immune function provides antioxidants and offers a tasty start to the day.

6. Spinach and Feta Egg Muffins:

   - Ingredients: Eggs, spinach, feta cheese, cherry tomatoes, garlic.

   - Pros: Packed with protein and portable, these egg muffins make for a tasty and satisfying breakfast.

7. Chia Pudding Parfait:

   - Ingredients: Chia seeds, almond milk, vanilla extract, Greek yogurt, forest fruit mixture.

   - Benefits: A nutrient- and fiber-rich custard parfait that offers omega-3 fatty acids from chia seeds and a blend of vitamins from berries.

8. Banana Nut Pancakes:

   - Ingredients: Whole grain flour, bananas, walnuts, almond milk, and cinnamon.

   - Benefits: Hearty and healthy pancakes with the natural sweetness of bananas and the crunch of walnuts for sustained energy.

9. Tropical Acai Bowl:

   - Ingredients: Acai puree, banana, mango, coconut water, granola, coconut flakes.

   - Benefits: A refreshing and tropical acai bowl providing antioxidants, vitamins and minerals for a lively start to the day.

10. Sweet potato and cabbage breakfast porridge:

   - Ingredients: Sweet potatoes, cabbage, eggs, red onion, garlic, olive oil.

   - Benefits: A savory, nutrient-dense breakfast cereal with the added benefits of vitamin A from sweet potatoes and the antioxidant power of kale.

Lunchtime Healing: Light and Nutritious Meals

Lunch is an opportunity for light and nutritious meals that will keep energy levels up throughout the day. Here we explore recipes designed to provide essential nutrients while being gentle on the digestive system. From vibrant salads to comforting soups, these midday healing options aim to promote overall well-being and resilience during your cancer journey.

1. Mediterranean Quinoa and Chickpea Salad:

   - Ingredients: Quinoa, chickpeas, cherry tomatoes, cucumber, feta cheese, olives, olive oil, lemon.

   - Benefits: A salad rich in protein and fiber with the

Mediterranean taste of olives and feta for a refreshing and nutritious lunch.

2. Light Lemon-Dill Chicken Soup:

   - Ingredients: Chicken, carrot, celery, dill, lemon, quinoa.

   - Benefits: Soothing and hydrating soup containing lean protein from chicken and digestive support from lemon and dill.

3. Spring rolls with avocado and shrimp:

   - Ingredients: Rice paper, shrimp, avocado, noodles, fresh herbs, peanut sauce.

- Benefits: A light and refreshing option rich in healthy fats from avocado and lean protein from shrimp combined with the freshness of herbs.

4. Caprese Zucchini Noodles:

   - Ingredients: Zucchini noodles, cherry tomatoes, fresh mozzarella, basil, balsamic glaze.

   - Benefits: A low-carb, nutrient-packed alternative to traditional pasta with the classic Caprese flavors of tomato, mozzarella and basil.

5. Broccoli and Spinach Detox Soup:

   - Ingredients: Broccoli, spinach, garlic, onion, vegetable broth.

   - Benefits: A nourishing and detoxifying soup with the cruciferous goodness of broccoli and the iron-rich properties of spinach.

6. Salad with tuna and white beans:

   - Ingredients: Canned tuna, white beans, cherry tomatoes, red onion, parsley, olive oil.

   - Benefits: Protein and satisfying tuna and white bean salad for sustained energy and a variety of nutrients.

7. Sweet Potato and Lentil Buddha Bowl:

   - Ingredients: Baked sweet potatoes, boiled lentils, cabbage, tahini dressing.

   - Benefits: A nutritious and balanced bowl containing sweet potatoes for complex carbohydrates and lentils for plant-based protein, topped with a creamy tahini dressing.

8. Cucumber Dill Greek Yogurt Chicken Wrap:

   - Ingredients: Grilled chicken, cucumber, Greek yogurt, dill, whole grain wrap.

- Benefits: A light and protein-rich wrap with a refreshing combination of cucumber and dill in a Greek yogurt dressing.

9. Spinach and strawberry salad with poppy seed dressing:

- Ingredients: Baby spinach, strawberries, feta cheese, almonds, poppy seed dressing.

- Benefits: A lively and antioxidant-rich salad combining the sweetness of strawberries, the earthiness of spinach and the crunch of almonds.

10. Miso-Ginger Tofu Stir-Fry:

- Ingredients: tofu, broccoli, paprika, peas, miso paste, ginger.

- Benefits: Plant-based and umami-rich stir-fried with tofu for protein and digestive support, miso and ginger.

Dinner Pleasures: Satisfying and Nutritious Dinners

Dinner is an opportunity to enjoy satisfying, nutrient-packed meals that promote healing and resilience. This explores recipes designed to deliver a soothing and nourishing end to the day. From hearty one-pot meals to delicious grilled dishes, these dinner treats are created to provide essential nutrients and help support a sense of well-being during the challenges of cancer treatment.

1. Pumpkin and lentil stew:

   - Ingredients: Butternut squash, lentils, carrots, celery, vegetable stock, turmeric.

   - Benefits: A hearty, fiber-rich stew with butternut squash for vitamins and lentils for plant-based protein.

2. Grilled Citrus Salmon with Herbed Quinoa:

   - Ingredients: Salmon fillets, citrus marinade, quinoa, fresh herbs.

- Benefits: A tasty dinner rich in omega-3 fatty acids with grilled salmon and nutrient-rich herb quinoa.

3. Cauliflower and Chickpea Curry:

- Ingredients: Cauliflower, chickpeas, tomatoes, coconut milk, curry spices.

- Benefits: Soothing and plant-based curry rich in fiber, protein and the anti-inflammatory effects of curry spices.

4. Bowl with roasted vegetables and brown rice:

  - Ingredients: Roasted
vegetables, brown rice, and tahini
dressing.

  - Benefits: A satisfying and
customizable bowl with the
nutritional benefits of roasted
vegetables and the healthy
goodness of brown rice.

5. Lemon-Garlic Herb Chicken
with Quinoa Pilaf:

  - Ingredients: Chicken breast,
lemon, garlic, mixed herbs,
quinoa.

  - Benefits: Savory and protein-
packed with lean chicken and
quinoa for a balanced and
satisfying dinner.

6. Sweet and Spicy Sautéed Tofu with Broccoli:

   - Ingredients: tofu, broccoli, soy sauce, honey, ginger, red pepper flakes.

   - Benefits: A plant-based and tasty stir-fry with tofu for protein and broccoli for added vitamins and minerals.

7. Mediterranean Stuffed Peppers:

   - Ingredients: Paprika, quinoa, chickpeas, tomatoes, feta cheese, olives.

   - Benefits: A colorful and nutrient-packed dinner with the

Mediterranean taste of olives, feta and quinoa.

8. Baked cod with tomatoes and olives:

   - Ingredients: Cod fillets, cherry tomatoes, olives, garlic, olive oil.

   - Benefits: A light variant rich in omega-3 with baked cod and a tasty tomato and olive taste.

9. Spaghetti pumpkin with pesto and cherry tomatoes:

   - Ingredients: Spaghetti pumpkin, homemade pesto, cherry tomatoes, pine nuts.

   - Advantages: A low-carb and nutritious alternative to traditional pasta with the lively taste of homemade pesto.

10. Black Bean and Veggie Enchiladas:

   - Ingredients: Black beans, peppers, corn, whole wheat tortillas, enchilada sauce.

   - Benefits: A satisfying and plant-based dinner with black beans for protein and a variety of vegetables for added nutrients.

Snacks for Sustainable Energy

Snacking plays a key role in maintaining energy levels and providing essential nutrients throughout the day, especially during the challenges of cancer treatment. This explores snacks designed to provide sustained energy, satisfy cravings and contribute to overall well-being. From protein-packed bites to refreshing fruit options, these snacks are created to be convenient, delicious and support a resilient, nourished body.

1. Trail mix for an energy boost:

   - Ingredients: Mixed nuts, seeds, dried fruit, and dark chocolate.

   - Benefits: Nutrient-rich portable snack with an energy-boosting combination of nuts, seeds and the sweetness of dried fruit and dark chocolate.

2. Greek yogurt parfait with fruit:

   - Ingredients: Greek yogurt, mixed berries, granola.

   - Benefits: A protein-rich and satisfying parfait offering the probiotic benefits of Greek yogurt and the natural sweetness of berries.

3. Hummus and vegetable sticks:

   - Ingredients: Hummus, carrot sticks, cucumber slices, pepper strips.

- Benefits: A snack rich in fiber and flavor containing hummus for protein and a variety of colorful vegetables for added nutrients.

4. Apple slices with almond butter:

   - Ingredients: apple slices, almond butter.

   - Benefits: A simple and balanced snack that provides the natural sweetness of apples and the satiating properties of almond butter.

5. Edamame and Sea Salt:

   - Ingredients: Edamame, sea salt.

- Benefits: A protein and salty snack containing edamame, providing vegetable protein and essential amino acids.

6. Cottage cheese with pineapple:

   - Ingredients: Cottage cheese, pieces of fresh pineapple.

   - Benefits: A protein-rich and refreshing snack combining the creaminess of cottage cheese with the sweetness of pineapple.

7. Dark Chocolate Nut Clusters:

   - Ingredients: Dark chocolate, mixed nuts.

   - Benefits: A satisfying and antioxidant-rich snack with a

combination of dark chocolate and nutritionally rich nuts.

8. Rice cake with avocado and cherry tomatoes:

   - Ingredients: Rice cake, avocado, cherry tomatoes, sea salt.

   - Benefits: A light and balanced snack offering heart-healthy fats from avocado and the freshness of cherry tomatoes.

9. Popcorn with turmeric and black pepper:

   - Ingredients: Popcorn, turmeric, black pepper.

   - Benefits: A tasty and antioxidant-rich snack with the anti-inflammatory properties of turmeric and the digestive effects of black pepper.

10. Smoothie with spinach and banana:

   - Ingredients: spinach, banana, Greek yogurt, almond milk.

   - Benefits: Nutrient-packed and hydrating snack in the form of a smoothie with the green goodness of spinach and the natural sweetness of banana.

Smoothies and Juices

In liquid nutrition, smoothies and juices offer a convenient and delicious way to deliver a concentrated dose of essential nutrients. This explores different formulas designed to provide hydration, vitamins and minerals, making them especially valuable during the challenges of cancer treatment. From vibrant fruit smoothies to nutrient-rich green juices, these drinks are created to promote overall well-being and offer a refreshing and nutritious experience.

1. Berry Blast Smoothie:

   - Ingredients: A mixture of berries (strawberries, blueberries, raspberries), banana, Greek yogurt, almond milk.

- Benefits: Antioxidant-rich and hydrating smoothie with mixed berries and protein support from Greek yogurt.

2. Green Goddess Detox Juice:

   - Ingredients: Cabbage, cucumber, green apple, celery, lemon, ginger.

   - Benefits: Cleansing and nourishing green juice with kale for vitamins and minerals and refreshing properties of cucumber and lemon.

3. Tropical Paradise Smoothie Bowl:

   - Ingredients: Pineapple, mango, banana, coconut water,

toppings (granola, coconut flakes).

   - Benefits: Tropical and hydrating smoothie bowl with pineapple and mango for a dose of vitamins and minerals.

4. Carrot-Orange Juice to Boost Immunity:

   - Ingredients: Carrot, orange, turmeric, ginger.

   - Benefits: Immune-boosting juice containing beta-carotene from carrots and the anti-inflammatory properties of turmeric and ginger.

5. Creamy Avocado Spinach Smoothie:

- Ingredients: Avocado, spinach, banana, almond milk, chia seeds.

- Benefits: Creamy and nutritious smoothie full of healthy fats from avocado and iron-rich spinach.

6. Antioxidant beet and berry juice:

- Ingredients: Beetroot, mixed berries, apple, lemon.

- Benefits: Antioxidant-rich juice with beets for detoxification and a blend of berries for a burst of flavor.

7. Peanut Butter Banana Protein Smoothie:

- Ingredients: Almond milk, protein powder, peanut butter, and banana.

- Benefits: Protein and satisfying smoothie with the nutty richness of peanut butter and potassium from bananas.

8. Cucumber Mint Cooler:

- Ingredients: cucumber, lime, honey, and mint leaves.

- Benefits: A refreshing and hydrating drink with cucumber and mint that provides a burst of flavor and potential digestive benefits.

9. Blueberry Almond Butter Smoothie:

- Ingredients: Blueberries, almond butter, Greek yogurt, almond milk.

   - Benefits: A creamy antioxidant-rich smoothie with the sweetness of blueberries and protein support from almond butter.

10. Hydrating Watermelon Juice:

   - Ingredients: Watermelon, basil leaves, lime.

   - Benefits: Hydrating and revitalizing juice with high water content in watermelon and refreshing aroma of basil.

These smoothies and juices are designed to be not only delicious and hydrating, but also packed with nutrients that support overall well-being during cancer treatment. Whether enjoyed as a quick and nutritious snack or incorporated into your diet, these drinks offer a wonderful way to stay hydrated and energized.

Chapter Five

Special Considerations

Navigating the nuances of an oncology diet requires attention to special considerations to address the unique needs and challenges that may arise during treatment. It provides guidance on how to adapt the Cancer Diet Cookbook to specific situations and considerations, and offers practical tips and recipes tailored to solve common problems.

1. Management of treatment side effects:

- Considerations: Addressing issues such as nausea, taste changes and difficulty swallowing.

- Tips: Explore gentle, easy-to-digest recipes like smooth soups, mildly flavored dishes, and cold options that may be more appealing during treatment.

2. Maintaining nutrient density:

- Considerations: Ensuring adequate intake of essential nutrients despite potential changes in appetite.

- Tips: Include nutrient-dense ingredients in meals and snacks and consider supplementation if recommended by health professionals.

3. Weight Management:

   - Considerations: Addressing weight loss or gain during treatment.

   - Tips: Adjusting portion sizes, incorporating calorie-dense foods, and focusing on balanced meals to support a healthy weight.

4. Hydration Challenges:

   - Considerations: Managing problems with water intake due to side effects of treatment.

   - Tips: Research hydrating foods, create flavored water with natural ingredients, and consider hydrating drinks like herbal teas.

5. Support of the immune system:

   - Considerations: Strengthening the immune system during treatment.

   - Tips: Include immune-boosting ingredients like garlic, ginger, and foods rich in vitamins C and D.

6. Oral Health:

   - Considerations: Addressing potential oral health problems during treatment.

- Tips: Choose soft and easy-to-chew foods, include soothing options like smoothies and soups, and maintain good oral hygiene.

7. Emotional well-being:

   - Considerations: Recognizing the emotional impact of cancer diagnosis and treatment.

   - Tips: Focus on comforting and familiar foods, incorporate mood-enhancing ingredients, and create a positive and receptive eating environment.

8. Adjustments for different diets:

   - Considerations: accommodating a range of

dietary requirements and preferences.

   - Tips: Offers substitutions and alternatives for common allergens or dietary preferences to make the cookbook accessible and adaptable for different needs.

9. Consultation with health professionals:

   - Considerations: It is important to seek advice from healthcare professionals.

   - Tips: Encourage readers to consult their healthcare team for personalized advice, especially regarding dietary changes during cancer treatment.

10. Family Friendly Adaptations:

   - Considerations: Adapting recipes to suit the tastes and preferences of family members.

   - Tips: Offers versatile recipes that can be adjusted to individual preferences, ensuring the cookbook is inclusive for families going through the cancer journey together.

Cooking for Convenience

Amidst the challenges of cancer treatment, finding comfort in food becomes a crucial aspect of overall well-being. This is dedicated to recipes that go beyond nutritional considerations, focusing on the emotional and comforting aspects of cooking. From hearty stews to comforting teas, these recipes are crafted to provide warmth, nourishment, and a sense of culinary comfort during difficult times.

1. Hearty chicken and vegetable stews:

   - Ingredients: Chicken, carrots, potatoes, onions, garlic, broth.

   - Purpose: A soothing and nourishing stew that brings warmth and familiarity.

2. Creamy Butternut Squash Risotto:

- Ingredients: Butternut
squash, Arborio rice, Parmesan
cheese, vegetable broth.

- Purpose: A creamy and
comforting risotto with the
sweetness of butternut squash.

3. Ginger-Turmeric Immunity
Tea:

- Ingredients: Fresh ginger,
turmeric, honey, lemon.

- Purpose: A soothing immune-
boosting tea that provides
comfort and warmth.

4. Classic Chicken Noodle Soup:

- Ingredients: Chicken,
noodles, carrots, celery, broth.

- Purpose: A timeless and familiar soup known for its soothing properties, ideal for easy digestion.

5. Baked Macaroni and Cheese:

   - Ingredients: Macaroni, cheese, milk, butter.

   - Purpose: Classic comfort food that brings enjoyment and familiarity to the table.

6. Mashed potatoes with garlic and rosemary:

   - Ingredients: Potatoes, garlic, rosemary, butter.

- Purpose: Creamy mashed potatoes with aromatic rosemary and garlic as a soothing side dish.

7. Chamomile-Lavender Relaxation Tea:

   - Ingredients: Chamomile tea bags, dried lavender, honey.

   - Purpose: A soothing and fragrant tea blend to promote relaxation and well-being.

8. Oatmeal with cinnamon and raisins:

   - Ingredients: Oatmeal, cinnamon, raisins, milk.

   - Purpose: A warm and nutritious bowl of oatmeal,

infused with the comforting flavor of cinnamon and raisins.

9. Roasted Garlic Tomato Soup:

   - Ingredients: Tomatoes, garlic, onions, basil, broth.

   - Purpose: A rich and tasty soup combining the sweetness of roasted tomatoes and spicy notes of garlic.

10. Dark Chocolate Avocado Mousse:

   - Ingredients: avocado, dark chocolate, honey.

   - Purpose: A decadent and nutritious dessert that provides a touch of indulgence.

Chapter Six

Meal Planning and Preparation

Effective meal planning and preparation are essential aspects of maintaining a well-balanced diet, especially during the challenges of cancer treatment. It focuses on practical strategies, tips and customizable meal plans to simplify the process for individuals and their caregivers. From organizing shopping lists to creating versatile recipes, this guide aims to empower readers to approach meal planning and preparation with confidence and ease.

1. Building a nutrient-rich pantry:

   - Instructions: Stock up on the necessary staples in the pantry.

   - Tips: Identify stable, nutrient-dense foods like whole grains, legumes, canned vegetables, and healthy oils.

2. Weekly meal planning:

   - Instructions: Organization of meals for a week in advance.

   - Tips: Plan balanced meals that include different food groups. Consider individual preferences, dietary restrictions, and energy levels when planning meals.

3. Creating Adaptable Recipes:

- Tutorial: Developing versatile recipes for different needs.

   - Tips: Create recipes that can be easily adjusted to suit taste preferences, dietary requirements and portion sizes. This flexibility helps adapt to changing appetites.

4. Batch cooking and freezing:

- Instructions: Streamlining meal preparation using batch cooking.

   - Tips: Make large batches of meals and freeze them in serving-size containers for convenient, ready-to-eat options.

5. Fast food rich in nutrients:

   - Instructions: Incorporating snacks that are easy to prepare.

   - Tips: Keep a selection of quick, nutrient-dense snacks like pre-cut veggies, yogurt, and nuts on hand for convenient, healthy options between meals.

6. Kitchen gadgets that save time:

   - Instructions: Use tools to speed up the cooking process.

   - Tips: Invest in kitchen gadgets like a slow cooker, instant pot or food processor to save time and effort when preparing meals.

7. Preparation for treatment side effects:

   - Guidelines: Adapting meal plans to potential side effects.

   - Tips: Anticipate and address potential changes in taste, appetite or digestion. Plan easy-to-digest and appealing options.

8. Collaboration in the kitchen:

   - Instructions: Involve family or friends in preparing food.

   - Tips: Share responsibilities in the kitchen to make meal preparation a shared and enjoyable experience. This can also promote a sense of support and connection.

9. Mindful Shopping Strategies:

- Directions: Make informed decisions at the grocery store.

- Tips: Give preference to fresh products, lean proteins and whole grains. To promote general health, choose foods that are high in nutrients.

10. Celebrating Food Diversity:

- Instructions: Exploring different cuisines and tastes.

- Tips: Adopt different recipes and ingredients to keep meals interesting and enjoyable. This approach can introduce new nutrients and flavors into the diet.

By offering practical guidance and customizable approaches, it aims to simplify meal planning and preparation for individuals and their caregivers. Through effective strategies and thoughtful choices, the goal is to make the experience of preparing and enjoying meals during cancer treatment a nutritious and manageable aspect of everyday life.

Support from Family and Friends

The support of family and friends is a vital part of coping with the challenges of the cancer journey. This focuses on fostering a support network and encouraging meaningful connections between individuals undergoing treatment and their loved ones. From communication strategies to practical ways to help, this guide aims to empower individuals facing cancer and those who want to offer support.

1. Open communication:

   - Instructions: Establish open and honest communication.

   - Tips: Encourage transparent conversations about feelings, needs and preferences. Create a platform where individuals feel comfortable expressing their thoughts.

2. Coordination of care:

   - Counseling: Coordinating support efforts among friends and family.

   - Tips: Create a central point of contact for updates and coordinate tasks such as food delivery, transportation and assistance with daily activities.

3. Practical help:

   - Guidance: Offering specific help with daily tasks.

   - Tips: Help with grocery shopping, meal preparation,

transportation to meetings and
other practical tasks to ease the
daily burden.

4. Emotional support:

   - Counseling: Providing
emotional reassurance and
companionship.

   - Tips: Offer to listen, engage in
activities that bring joy, and
provide emotional support during
challenging times.

5. Flexibility and adaptability:

   - Guidelines: Remain flexible
and adapt to changing needs.

   - Tips: Respond to the evolving
needs of individuals facing

cancer. Be willing to adjust plans and support based on the current situation.

6. Respecting boundaries:

   - Counseling: Recognizing and respecting personal boundaries.

   - Tips: Keep in mind that an individual needs space and privacy. Communicate openly about what types of support are most helpful and when.

7. Celebrating milestones:

   - Guidelines: Acknowledging and celebrating successes.

   - Tips: Recognize small and significant milestones on the road to cancer. Celebrate successes, whether they're related to treatment progress or personal victories.

8. Facilitation of social contacts:

   - Guidelines: Encourage social interactions and community engagement.

   - Tips: Help facilitate social contacts by organizing small get-togethers or outings that give individuals the opportunity to engage with a supportive community.

9. Provision of information and resources:

- Instructions: Offer useful resources and information.

  - Tips: Share reliable and relevant information about cancer treatment, dietary considerations and available support resources. Help gather information that can help make decisions.

10. Permanent support after treatment:

  - Counselling: Ongoing support after the treatment phase.

  - Tips: Be aware that support may be needed even after a period of active treatment. Continue to check in, offer assistance, and provide emotional support as needed.

Beyond the Plate

While nutrition and dietary choices are essential components of the cancer journey, there are many aspects beyond what's on the plate that contribute to overall well-being. This study examines a holistic approach to health that includes lifestyle factors, emotional support, and self-care strategies to enhance quality of life during and after cancer treatment. This guide aims to empower individuals to take a comprehensive approach to their health, from mindfulness practices to staying active.

1. Mindfulness and meditation:

   - Practice: Bringing mindfulness into daily existence.

   - Tips: Explore mindfulness meditation techniques, deep breathing exercises, or mindful eating practices to cultivate a sense of calm and presence.

2. Physical activity and movement:

   - Exercise: Engaging in appropriate physical activity.

   - Tips: Consult with health professionals to determine

appropriate exercises. Include gentle activities such as walking, yoga or tai chi to promote physical well-being.

3. Emotional well-being and counseling:

   - Practice: Addressing emotional health through counseling.

   - Tips: Consider seeking professional counseling or therapy to manage the emotional issues associated with a cancer diagnosis and treatment.

4. Quality sleep habits:

   - Exercise: Prioritizing quality sleep.

- Tips: Create a calming bedtime routine, create a comfortable sleep environment, and stick to a consistent sleep schedule to promote restful sleep.

5. Stress Reduction Techniques:

   - Exercise: Implementing stress reduction strategies.

   - Tips: Explore stress reduction techniques such as deep breathing, progressive muscle relaxation, or engaging in hobbies and activities that bring joy.

6. Social ties:

   - Practice: Cultivating meaningful social ties.

- Tips: Stay connected with friends and family. Join support groups or get involved in community activities to create a network of understanding and supportive individuals.

7. Creative Expression:

   - Exercise: Use of creative outlets.

   - Tips: Explore creative activities such as art, writing or music to express emotions, find solace and engage in activities that bring joy.

8. Spiritual well-being:

   - Exercise: Caring for spiritual connection.

  - Tips: Engage in practices that align with personal beliefs, whether through prayer, meditation, or connecting with nature, to promote spiritual well-being.

9. Setting personal goals:

  - Practice: Making meaningful and practical goals.

  - Tips: Set achievable goals that contribute to a sense of accomplishment and purpose. Celebrate progress, no matter how small.

10. Continuing Education and Advocacy:

- Practice: Stay informed and advocate for personal health.

- Tips: Continue to educate yourself about cancer survival, treatment options, and lifestyle choices. Advocate for personal health needs with health professionals.